ABOUT THE AUTHOR

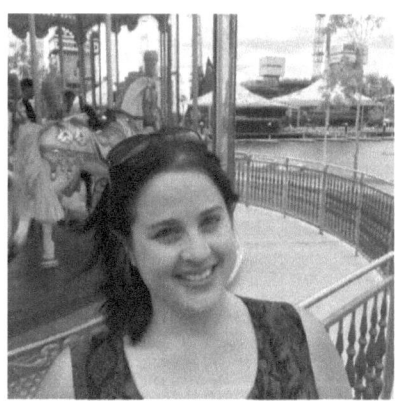

Thanks so much for purchasing "Magnificent Magnesium". My name is Jennifer Matthews and I am also known as Naturopath Jen. I am a qualified Naturopath, Law of Attraction Practitioner, Spiritual Life Coach and Self-Empowerment Educator. I have spent the last decade researching and spending thousands of dollars on my own personal development, as well as previously hosting multiple podcasts and blogs in the areas of health, wellness, mindset and spirituality.

I am now the founder and developer of the "Superconscious Success" Platform and the "Ask Naturopath Jen" Brand.

To learn more about myself and my journey (as it is quite an extensive read), please visit my personal site: http://www.spiritualcoachjenmatthews.com, where I delve into my purpose for writing these books and creating these brands and all the products/services (both free and paid) that can help you.

ABOUT THE BOOK

Magnificent Magnesium is the first book in the ANJ Series because it is a mineral that I absolutely love and have a lot of faith in. With so many people suffering from a magnesium deficiency and not even knowing it, I thought it was definitely important information to get out there for those looking at optimising their health.

OTHER BOOKS IN THIS SERIES

(All Available in Amazon under Naturopath Jen)

MSM Uncovered
Healing with Astaxanthin
Beginners Guide to Healing Leaky Gut Syndrome
The Acne Solution

DISCLAIMER

Please note that the information given in this book is for informational purposes only and is not intended to replace the advice of your health practitioner. If you experience symptoms that you are concerned with, please refer to your practitioner for further information...

****

SECTION 1 – ALL ABOUT MAGNESIUM

****

Chapter #1 - Magnesium Basics

****

What is Magnesium?

Magnesium is a vital mineral that is crucial for many functions in the body, including over 300 different enzymatic activities, including such things as:

- Energy production;

- Oxygen uptake;

- Central nervous system function;

- Balance of electrolyte levels;

- Glucose metabolism, and

- Muscle activity.

About 65% of the magnesium in our body is contained in the bones and teeth and the bones hold onto the magnesium as a reservoir for when it is needed. The remaining 35% of it will be contained within the blood, fluid and other tissues, and like potassium, most of it is found within the cells.

Magnesium, just like potassium, is an intracellular nutrient which occurs in very low levels in the blood, with the normal range being 1.7-2.4 m/Eq/liter. Not only does it activate enzymes important for protein and carbohydrate metabolism, but it is also required for DNA production and function.

Optimization of magnesium is essential as it modulates the electrical potential across the cell membranes, therefore allowing the nutrients to pass back and forth. Without this happening, the ability for it to convert the phosphate molecule to ATP (energy) will be limited.

Symptoms of Magnesium Deficiency

There are many different symptoms and conditions you may be experiencing which could indicate a deficiency in magnesium:

- Aggression;
- Anxiety;
- Brain Fog;
- Chronic Back Pain;
- Chronic Fatigue Syndrome;
- Chronic Stress;
- Constipation;
- Depression;
- Difficulty Swallowing;
- Dysmenorrhea;
- Fatigue;
- Fibromyalgia;
- Heart Palpitations;
- Hypertension (High Blood Pressure);
- Insomnia;
- Involuntary Eye Movements/Twitching;
- Kidney Stones;
- Loss of Appetite;
- Memory Loss;
- Menstrual Cramps;
- Migraines;
- Muscle Cramps;
- Muscular Pain;
- Nerve Problems;
- Noise Sensitivity;
- Osteoporosis;
- Panic Attacks;
- Poor Nail Growth;
- Sugar Cravings;
- Tendonitis.

Causes and Risk Factors for Magnesium Deficiency

There are many different factors that can contribute to a magnesium deficiency, apart from poor food quality. These include:

Alcohol Consumption

As alcohol increases urine production, it also increases excretion of magnesium. To learn more, check out Chapter 2 (FAQ's) on how alcohol affects magnesium.

Mercury fillings

If you have amalgam fillings at all then you may be surprised to know that these fillings can be causing a deficiency in magnesium. Even if you have silver amalgams and not pure mercury fillings, it is interesting to note that even silver fillings have 50% mercury.

Exposure to mercury has been shown to impede magnesium absorption, so if it is possible to remove the mercury fillings then you will find an increase in your magnesium levels.

However, please note that it is not a good idea to have this done by just any dentist. You really need to go to a holistic dentist who is specialized in removing these fillings as they can release a lot of toxins and heavy metals into your bloodstream if a proper detox is not done first (make sure you are taking plenty of magnesium during this detox as it is important for the liver).

There is plenty of information on the internet regarding this so read up a little more on it if this is something you are wanting to do.

Fluoride

Like with mercury, exposure to fluoride impairs magnesium absorption in the intestines. It has been shown that by supplementing with magnesium you can offset its toxicity.

Therefore, my suggestion would be to try to avoid fluoride as much as possible by investing in a good quality water filter/shower filter and if you choose to, avoid fluoridated toothpastes and then take magnesium supplements to offset the potential toxicities.

Coffee Consumption

Drinking coffee is able to affect the levels of magnesium in your body by inhibiting absorption in the intestines. Although it does not directly deplete the magnesium levels in the body, its inhibitory effect can lead to a gradual decrease in magnesium levels.

If you are going to drink coffee it is a good idea to make sure you take magnesium supplementation and/or make sure you eat plenty of magnesium rich foods. To get a full listing, you can read page "24" on Nutritional Sources of Magnesium.

Birth Control Pills

There are many side effects that birth control pills can cause, including nutrient depletion. Not only do they deplete the body of magnesium, but they also deplete the body of Vitamin B2, Vitamin B6, Vitamin B12, Folic Acid, Vitamin C and Zinc.

If you are currently on birth control pills, it is advisable you consider supplementing with the nutrients that are depleted (including magnesium).

Excessive Stress

Studies have shown that an extremely stressful experience or a series of lower levels of stress depletes the body of magnesium. Stress hormone production requires high levels of magnesium and therefore stress can lead to a deficiency.

Not only can stress lead to a depletion of magnesium, but magnesium supplementation can help you handle your stress a lot better, therefore reducing the chance of the magnesium deficiency caused by excessive stress.

Sweat loss during Exercise

Studies have shown that strenuous exercise increases urinary and sweat losses which may increase magnesium requirements by 10-20%.

Soft Drink Consumption

In the intestines, the phosphoric acid found in soft drinks combines with magnesium to form magnesium phosphate, an insoluble type of magnesium that is excreted through the faeces.

Drinking soft drinks high in phosphates causes an imbalance of the two minerals, phosphorus and magnesium and therefore interferes with the body's ability to absorb not only magnesium, but also calcium and iron.

Excess Calcium

Consuming extra calcium is known to deplete magnesium levels, as well as increase the body's need for magnesium. Without adequate magnesium, calcium will not be able to be utilized, which makes it virtually useless.

Poor Absorption Due to Low Stomach Acid

When your stomach acid is low it reduces your body's ability to break down food and supplements to its usable form, including Magnesium. If you are suffering from low stomach acid, it may be an idea to supplement with a hydrochloric acid supplement.

Small Intestine Issues

If you are suffering from issues with the small intestine, such as GI infections, inflammatory bowel disease, radiation induced gastroenteritis, severe diarrhea and/or familial malabsorption syndromes, then a deficiency can also occur.

Overactive thyroid

Studies have shown that an excessive amount of thyroid hormones, as seen in hyperthyroidism decreases the absorption of magnesium, therefore making it more likely that people who are hyperthyroid are deficient in magnesium.

Poor Soil Quality

Another reason so many people are deficient in magnesium is because of the poor soil quality where our vegetables are grown and where synthetic fertilizers are used, that contain no magnesium at all.

Types of Supplemental Magnesium

When considering what type of magnesium, you should take it is important that you take into account the absorb-ability of it, what form you would like to take it in and also what effects you are hoping to receive.

Supplemental Magnesium is able to be absorbed in 3 different ways:

- Trans-dermal Magnesium;
- Epsom Salts; and/or
- Supplemental Powders and Pills.
- Trans-dermal Magnesium (Magnesium Chloride)

Trans-dermal delivery has been shown to be the most effective way of absorbing magnesium into the body. Unless you have kidney issues, your body will excrete any magnesium that is not required, therefore toxicity is very rare, even with oral supplementation.

However, Trans-dermal application is the safest and most effective form of application and it has been shown to increase the body's magnesium levels up to 5 times faster than oral supplementation.

As this magnesium is applied to the skin it avoids processing by the digestive system and kidneys, which prevents the laxative effects of other magnesium's. It also means that by using Trans-dermal magnesium instead of supplemental magnesium you are still able to absorb it even when you have digestive issues.

Although magnesium supplements are contraindicated in people with kidney issues, Trans-dermal magnesium is still able to be used as it does not have to filter through the kidneys.

Magnesium chloride is found in good quality himalayan sea salt and is also found in special flakes that you can get from health food shops or even via amazon. I have set up a special section on my site that you can go to in order to see a great selection of magnesium products that you can choose from. This link is supplied in the Conclusion.

Trans-dermal magnesium can be found in a bottle which you spray onto your skin and rub in. I use this magnesium regularly, especially as I am dealing with the aches and pains associated with my autoimmune condition – Hashimoto's Thyroiditis. It relieves leg pain quite quickly.

In fact, I am going to give you a personal story which will show you how remarkable this Trans-dermal magnesium is.

The other night, I was putting my 10-year-old adorable daughter Amelia to bed when she started crying and showed a complete expression of pain on her face. After asking what was wrong, she proceeded to tell me that one of her legs was in excruciating pain and that it felt heaps worse than "growing pains". She cried for about 1/2 an hour until I remembered I had some magnesium chloride flakes in the cupboard.

We both went and hopped in a bath full of these flakes, and then she told me that her leg was feeling better but still a bit sore. I then went and found my Trans-dermal magnesium spray that I had and rubbed it into her leg. Within 10 minutes of doing this, the pain had diminished so much she was able to sleep comfortably, and her leg was all better the next day.

I do have one caution however. If you are indeed deficient in magnesium you may find that your skin will be prickly, itchy and burning a little. I find that after about 5-10 minutes that feeling will disappear and you will start to feel a lot better. If however you are not able to tolerate it, then dilute it first. It is often a good idea to do a skin test first and put a little on a small patch of skin to see if you have any reaction to that prior to covering a larger section.

Now, I have some good news. No longer do you have to pay for Trans-dermal spray anymore, you are able to make it yourself as long as you have some magnesium chloride flakes.

Any health food store should be able to provide you with these flakes, otherwise see the links in my conclusion to see where you can get them:

Ingredients/Supplies

1 cup of magnesium chloride flakes;

1 cup of distilled or filtered water, free of chlorine, fluoride and toxic chemicals;

Cast iron, a stainless steel or a glass saucepan (not aluminium).

Methods

- Bring the filtered/distilled water to a boil;
- Add the magnesium flakes until they are dissolved;
- Remove this solution from the heat and let it cool.
- Once this mixture has cooled, transfer it to a spray bottle to use.

Please Note: 8 sprays of this magnesium oil spray delivers about 100mg of elemental magnesium to the skin. For maximal absorption, try rubbing it into your torso.

Epsom Salts (Magnesium Sulfate)

Ingested Orally, Magnesium Sulfate is not easily absorbed. However, studies have shown that when it is absorbed through the skin, as is the case with Epsom Baths, it is very effective at increasing your level of magnesium.

By doing this, not only are you absorbing the magnesium through the skin which has a whole host of benefits, but it also absorbs the sulfate through the skin too. Sulfate has been found to play an important role in the formation of brain tissue, joint proteins and also the proteins that line the walls of the digestive tract.

Both the magnesium and the sulfate together are known to stimulate detoxification.

Epsom Salts are incredibly inexpensive to purchase, and I have included some amazon links in my store at http://www.asknaturopathjen.com/store

or else you can go to your local drug store and they will most likely have some you can purchase.

If you already have magnesium chloride flakes though, you can use them in the bath too. Try and bathe regularly in this so as to increase your magnesium levels.

Supplemental Powders and Pills

There are many different types of magnesium that you will find in the supplements you are taking. If you are considering supplementing your diet with magnesium, there are some factors you should take into account.

You should consider them based on their availability, their absorb-ability and their purpose. Therefore, I have listed the magnesium types, from most absorbable to least absorbable so you know what to look for when finding the right supplement for you.

#1 - Magnesium Taurate

This is best for those with cardiovascular issues, as it is known to prevent arrythmias and protect the heart from previous damage caused by heart attacks. It is easily absorbed and contains no laxative properties.

#2 - Magnesium Malate

If you are suffering from fatigue, this is the best form of magnesium to be taking. It is highly soluble.

#3 - Magnesium Glycinate

To correct an ongoing deficiency, this magnesium may be your choice as it has no laxative properties and it is also one of the most bio-available and absorb-able forms.

#4 - Magnesium Orotate

This is the most effective form of magnesium as it is a combination of magnesium and orotic acid. it has been shown to penetrate cell membranes, therefore enabling the effective delivery of the magnesium to the inner layers of the mitochondria and nucleus.

Not only do people use it for the magnesium content, but they also may use it for the orotic acid content instead. This acid is used for improving athletic performance and endurance, as well as for heart health.

The only problem with this type of magnesium is that it is so pricey, which is why so many supplements use magnesium aspartate instead.

#5 - Magnesium Aspartate

This form of magnesium has an absorption rate of up to 70% which makes it one of the most absorbed types of magnesium. It also has a very high retention rate in the blood after absorption, unlike other forms which are quickly excreted.

However, please note that there are differing opinions on whether this supplement is good or not due to the "Aspartate" side of it. If you would like to know more you can research it further and see what you think.

#6 - Magnesium Citrate

Like with the aspartate, this form of magnesium is very well absorbed, however it is pricy so you will find most companies will use aspartate as it is much cheaper to make.

#7 - Magnesium Lactate

Although this type of magnesium should be avoided by those with kidney issues, it has a higher level of absorption than magnesium oxide does.

#8 - Magnesium Phosphate

This type of magnesium is OK, but it is very rarely found available, except in tissue salts for homeopathic remedies. Often when a cheaper supplement is created, this type of magnesium will be thrown in to make it at least semi absorbable.

#9 - Magnesium Oxide/Magnesium Hydroxide

These two types of magnesium are not to be used for a very long time as they are actually antacids and laxatives. You will find these types of magnesium in cheap supplements as they are inexpensive to produce.

Oxide is basically 60% magnesium and Hydroxide is 40%. However, both of them are so poorly absorbed and they end up staying in the bowels instead. Magnesium Hydroxide (also known as Milk of Magnesia) will often be used if somebody has low stomach acid.

However, remember that magnesium requires stomach acid to be able to be absorbed and therefore the low stomach acid is just going to cause the magnesium to not be absorbed anyway.

#10 - Magnesium Carbonate

Carbonate has a strong laxative effect so although it has a 30% bio-availability rate, it is not the ideal magnesium type to take. It is commonly known as chalk and is used by gymnasts, rock climbers and weight lifters.

Best Time to take Magnesium

In order to get the most out of your magnesium supplementation, it is best to take it between meals or at bedtime, as it requires an acidic stomach environment for optimal absorption. Try to avoid taking it with foods that are high in calcium or phosphorus as they can both compete with magnesium.

Optimal Intakes of Magnesium

When we are talking about how much magnesium we should be taking, there is a difference between the RDA levels of Magnesium and the levels of magnesium that are optimal.

The RDA recommends 350mg/day for males, 280mg/day for females and 350mg/day for pregnant and lactating women. However, the optimal level is actually as high as 600-800mg per day.

Every person is different, so it requires you to test it yourself and see what your optimal level is before you start feeling the benefits. However, I don't just recommend that you take supplementation, but also that you incorporate magnesium rich foods, such as leafy green vegetables, nuts and fish so as to up your level.

Toxicity of Magnesium

This mineral is an extremely safe mineral and can be taken in very high doses, as it tends to be excreted when taken in excess.

However, there are a few pointers you should take into consideration:

• If you have kidney disease or kidney issues, use Trans-dermal magnesium or Epsom bath salts instead, because your kidneys are required to filter out the excess magnesium.

• If you take too high a quantity of certain types of magnesium, there is a side effect of diarrhea. If this happens, taper back your intake until the diarrhea stops.

• The risk of toxicity increases if your calcium levels are low, so make sure that you have a sufficient amount of calcium in your diet as well. The ratio of calcium to magnesium should be 2:1 for optimal health. When your calcium levels are insufficient, and you take extra magnesium it can cause a depression of the central nervous system, leading to muscle weakness, fatigue, sleepiness, and can even lead to death.

• It is also not recommended to take magnesium supplementation when you have myasthenia gravis, atrial fibrillation or a high level of magnesium (very rare).

Testing for Magnesium

As magnesium lives within the cells and not in the blood, blood tests are not the most accurate way of measuring magnesium levels. Most of the magnesium in our body is stored within the cells and not the blood itself. Therefore, blood magnesium levels can be misleading. In fact, people with low levels of magnesium have still been found to have normal blood levels, so serum blood tests are not reliable.

However, for reference sake, the normal range for the serum blood levels are: 1.5 - 2.5 mEq/liter.

Instead of serum blood levels, there are a number of other ways that you can test for your magnesium levels:

#1 TEST - Going By Signs of Deficiency

It is in my opinion, and many other people's opinions that magnesium tests are not necessary. Due to the fact that your magnesium levels can change far too quickly, and everybody's ideal amount is different depending on their specific needs, the best way to see if you have an issue with magnesium is to start taking it, either orally or trans-dermally and see if your symptoms improve.

As it is generally a non-toxic supplement (check out toxicity section for further information) it is not going to hurt you to do an N=1 experiment and test your symptoms. However, if you do want to get a test done, there are a couple of tests you can do.

Hair/Mineral Analysis

I find that hair and mineral analysis is a great test to have done if you are wanting to test for macro-mineral, trace mineral and toxic metal deficiencies and excesses. It is a safe, non-invasive test that measures the minerals deposited in the cells and interstitial spaces of the hair over a 2-3 month period.

Although it does not give you an indication of other tissues of the body it may be a place to start because if you are deficient in the hair you are likely to be deficient in other tissues too.

A Hair Analysis Report shows the balance of your minerals such as magnesium, calcium, potassium and salt.

There are generally 15 trace minerals that are tested with this hair analysis:

- Calcium (ca);
- Magnesium (mg);
- Sodium (na);
- Potassium (k);
- Copper (cu);
- Zinc (zn);
- Phosphorus (p);
- Iron (fe);
- Manganese (mn);
- Chromium (cr);
- Selenium (se);
- Boron (b);
- Cobalt (co);
- Molybdenum (mo); and
- Sulfur (s).

The measurement of each of these minerals will be finely calibrated so that you can compare the levels of minerals against each other.

But before you go and just start supplementing because the report says you are low in something, you need to understand there are 2 different types of mineral deficiencies that are shown in these reports:

Absolute Mineral Deficiency - You are actually deficient in this mineral and it is typically due to decreased absorption and retention or not getting enough of it in the diet.

Relative Mineral Deficiency - This is when you have a deficiency of a mineral, relative to another mineral. Even if you are not deficient in that mineral it will show up as deficient because you have an excess of another one. Magnesium is a good example of this. If you have an excess of calcium, your magnesium levels will show up as deficient even though they are normal, because relative to calcium, your magnesium is not optimal.

Because we are trying to balance out the minerals in your body, especially in regards to calcium and magnesium, you may find the report recommends you take magnesium if your calcium is excessively high so that you can get the balance back in check, even if the magnesium seems high to start with.

Exa Test / Sublingual Epithelial Test

Although relatively new, this test seems to be one that is promising in regards to testing for your magnesium levels.

It is a reliable non-invasive procedure that measures the dynamic intracellular mineral electrolyte levels. This test provides information that is not available through blood or serum tests and takes the sample from the epithelial tissue in the mouth in a simple 60 second swab at the doctor's office.

The EXA test will offer you tissue evaluations for not only magnesium, but also phosphorus, calcium, sodium, potassium and chloride.

To read up more on EXA and find out where it is available, you can go to http://www.exatest.com.

Nutritional Sources of Magnesium

It is always best to try to get the magnesium from your diet prior to starting supplementation. Once you have adapted your diet to include high magnesium foods and taken into account all the strategies you need to adopt to make sure that you are absorbing as much magnesium as possible (check out my summary checklist" at the back of the book for these strategies) then you can consider implementing supplementation.

In terms of nutrition, the highest sources of magnesium include:

- Nuts, such as almonds and brazil nuts;
- Seeds, like pumpkin and sunflower;
- Fish, such as tuna;
- Raw Cacao;
- Dark, green leafy vegetables such as kale and spinach.

There are many sources of magnesium, with the highest level coming from dark, leafy green vegetables (due to the chlorophyll content) and seafood. Other sources include nuts, seeds and legumes, as well as grains. However, the magnesium found in grains are not absorbed due to the phytic acid. This phytic acid causes it to be eliminated rather than absorbed.

Also, when you boil your vegetables remember that the magnesium is leached into the water and so if you do use this form of cooking, make sure you make use of the water and/or steam the vegetables instead.

On top of that, if you are trying to get your magnesium from high oxalic acid foods (such as spinach and chard) then you may not be absorbing as much, because like with phytic acid, it causes the magnesium to be eliminated rather than absorbed.

Supplements that should be taken with Magnesium

Vitamin D

Because of the fact that Vitamin D actually uses magnesium to convert the vitamin d to its active form in the body, it is crucially important to take vitamin D and magnesium together.

Sometimes, when somebody takes Vitamin D, they may experience certain side effects. However, what they are experiencing is most often more a deficiency in magnesium than a toxicity of Vitamin D.

Vitamin C

Taking Vitamin C with your magnesium may help your body absorb it more efficiently.

Supplements to avoid taking with Magnesium

On top of supplements that should be taken with your Magnesium, there are some that you should avoid taking at the same time as your magnesium, as they fight with magnesium to be absorbed into the body. Therefore, the following supplements should be taken at a different time in the day than the magnesium, at least a couple of hours apart.

- Iron;
- Phosphorus;
- Manganese;
- Copper;
- Calcium.

Medications/Supplements that can interfere with how well you absorb Magnesium...

Cisplatin

A common drug used by cancer patients with their chemotherapy regime. Approximately 90% of patients taking this drug will need to also take an IV of Magnesium in order to prevent this deficiency.

Cyclosporine

A common drug used to treat hypertension. When somebody is taking this drug, a magnesium replacement may be necessary. An interesting study was done on an animal model showing that oral magnesium reduces the toxicity of this drug, even when the dietary intake of magnesium was normal.

Diuretics (loop and thiazide)

Use of diuretics is the most frequent cause of depleted magnesium levels.

Ethanol

Also known as alcohol, this substance has been shown to decrease levels of magnesium in the body.

Gentamicin Antibiotic

This is often used to treat serious bacterial infections. Studies have shown that even after as little as a week of being on this antibiotic, it is enough to cause a serious magnesium deficiency, as well as the associated hypo-calcemia (low calcium levels) and hypo-kalemia (low potassium levels).

Zinc

If you are taking zinc supplementation, then you should also take magnesium supplements as the intestinal absorption of magnesium is decreased in people taking oral zinc.

Medications, whose bioavailabilities are reduced by taking oral magnesium...

- Diclofenac;
- Diflusinol;
- Indomethasin;
- Naproxen;
- Quinidine;
- Levothyroxine;
- Quinolone Antibiotics;
- Tetracycline; and
- Related Antibiotics.

Chapter #2 - FAQS

****

Is it safe to take Magnesium During Pregnancy?

As mentioned above, apart from the few situations when supplementation should never be taken, magnesium is a very safe supplement, and is also considered essential during pregnancy.

When you are pregnant your requirements for magnesium increase and although the minimum required amount is 300mg per day, studies have shown that generally pregnant women only get 100mg from food per day, as well as 100mg from their supplementation and this leaves a deficiency of at least 100mg.

Due to the fact that there is an increased requirement of magnesium during pregnancy (because of the additional needs of magnesium with the growing baby) and the additional stress on the body with the pregnant mum, it is actually likely that you will require even more than that.

A deficiency of magnesium in the pregnant mother can be extremely dangerous, causing pre-eclampsia and toxemia, amongst other things. On a personal note, when I was pregnant with my first-born child, my son Jayman, I suffered from an extreme case of pre-eclampsia causing me to be admitted to hospital on and off for 2 weeks. I lived in Germany at the time and they were very efficient when it came to treating this issue. I was immediately placed on an IV of magnesium until my blood pressure had gone down.

Even if you don't get to this stage as a pregnant woman, there are other symptoms that may be experienced in the early stages of magnesium deficiency, such as migraines, headaches, back pain, muscle cramps, constipation, irritability, muscle tightness and even insomnia.

Although it is preferable to get your magnesium requirement from foods, the poor soil quality and excess consumption of processed foods in today's society makes this next to impossible. Therefore, supplementation is often a requirement. Have you ever thought of transdermal magnesium during pregnancy.

Now, in regards to the baby, magnesium supplementation is useful for the baby and has been shown to have a beneficial effect on fetal growth. They have shown that how a baby sleeps once they are born can be greatly influenced by how much magnesium has been passed to the baby during pregnancy.

Another reason for possibly taking magnesium during pregnancy is that studies have shown it can lead to higher birth weights, a decrease in the incidence of premature birth, a decrease in cerebral palsy and fewer neurological problems in the babies that have gone through an extremely traumatic birth.

Studies have shown that the highest dosage given to a pregnant lady that was magnesium deficient is 360mg per day and generally only during the second and third trimesters. Therefore, it has not been studied at higher levels and so if you feel you need more than this, it is advisable to check with your physician first.

Is Magnesium beneficial for athletes?

There have been numerous studies out there showing that magnesium can be beneficial for athletes or people that exercise regularly. Not only is it incredibly important for optimal energy production but it is also responsible for the production of ATP, the cells source of energy.

A scientific study on magnesium actually found that female endurance athletes who took magnesium supplements were able to run at a greater intensity for a longer time.

Also, if you are somebody that suffers from muscle cramps, you may be lacking in valuable electrolytes, such as sodium, magnesium and potassium. Adding these electrolytes back in can stop the muscle cramping and therefore make you a lot more effective with your exercise.

Magnesium is very important for cellular repair so if you are deficient in magnesium, your muscles will not be able to effectively repair themselves and so your rate of muscle growth will be slowed won considerably. Therefore, magnesium is shown as being necessary for recovery.

Finally, to optimally perform as an athlete, it is necessary to be properly hydrated. This means that not only should you make sure that you are drinking plenty of water but that you are getting enough electrolytes to replace the ones lost during intense exercise. As many athletes are magnesium deficient, it is often a good idea to supplement.

How Important is Magnesium for the Elderly?

Elderly people are at the greatest risk of suffering from hypomagnesemia, due to the fact that cardiovascular and heart issues become more common as you age and you find elderly people seem to take more diuretics than others. As shown above, diuretics are a serious contraindication with sustaining optimal magnesium levels.

How does alcohol and alcoholism affect magnesium levels?

As alcohol excretes magnesium through the urine by as much as 260% and this generally occurs within minutes of ingesting the alcohol, it is critically important that people consuming excess alcohol must take magnesium supplementation.

With chronic alcohol use, body stores of magnesium will become depleted. There are many reasons for this:

- Inadequate intake of magnesium;
- Starvation ketosis;
- Vomiting and/or Diarrhea; and
- Urinary Excretion.

Therefore, the effects of the chronic alcoholism are:

- Negative magnesium balance;
- Decreased plasma levels of magnesium;
- Decreased magnesium levels in cerebrospinal fluid, as well as muscle biopsies; and
- Development of magnesium responsive hypo-calcemia.

****

SECTION 2 – RESEARCH

****

Chapter #3 – ADD/ADHD

****

ADHD is a chronic condition where persistent inattention, hyperactivity and at times impulsivity are common features. This condition begins in childhood and often continues into adulthood.

Magnesium has been found to be helpful in treating children with Attention Deficit Disorder and Attention Deficit Hyperactivity Disorder. There are a number of ways that this works:

Relaxes The Mind

As the body uses magnesium to facilitate the sending of messages throughout the central nervous system, it is also used to calm the mind of children with hyperactivity disorders. They have found that kids who have sufficient amounts of magnesium in their body are able to think clearer and concentrate better. This mineral is also a requirement for the production of serotonin, which is an important neurotransmitter that provides a feeling of calm and well-being and therefore low levels of this neurotransmitter is associated with irritability, moodiness and depression.

Relaxes The Body

Just like with the mind, magnesium is a requirement for the relaxation of the muscle fibers and without this mineral, muscle cramping, muscle twitches and muscle spasms are common. Ensuring kids have a sufficient level of this nutrient will also give them the greater chance of reducing the hyperactivity.

Research Study #1 - "Magnesium Supplementation on ADHD in Children"

Starobrat-Hermelin B et al, "The effects of Magnesium Physiological Supplementation on Hyperactivity in Children with Attention Deficit Hyperactivity Disorder (ADHD). Positive Response to Magnesium Oral Loading Test", Magnesium Research, 1997

This study consisted of 50 ADHD hyperactive children, all aged between 7 and 12 years who had a recognized magnesium deficiency in the blood as well as in the hair.

In the study group there were 50 children who took 200mg per day over a 6-month period. Of these children, 30 of the children showed coexisting disorders specific to the developmental age and the other 20 showed disruptive behaviour.

In the control group it consisted of 25 children with ADHD and magnesium deficiency who were not treated with magnesium during the 6-month period. 15 of these children showed coexisting disorders specific to the developmental age and the other 10 showed disruptive behaviour.

After the 6-month period, they concluded that the children taking the magnesium had a significant reduction in hyperactivity symptoms than those that didn't.

Research Study #2 – Vitamin D and Magnesium Supplementation in Children with ADHD.

Hemamy M et al, "Effect of Vitamin D and Magnesium Supplementation on Behavior Problems in Children with Attention-Deficit Hyperactivity Disorder", Int J Prev Med, 2020.

This study was a double blind, randomized controlled clinical trial on 66 children with Attention Deficit Hyperactivity Disorder in Iran in 2016.

These children were randomly allocated to receive both Vitamin D (50,000IU per week) and Magnesium (6mg/kg/day) Supplements OR Placebo for a period of 8 weeks.

After 8 weeks, both Vitamin D and Magnesium increased significantly in the intervention group compared to placebo.

Although these supplements had no significant effect on psychosomatic scores, it did effect conduct problems, social problems and anxiety/shy scores.

Chapter 4 – Anxiety/Depression

****

Anxiety: *Feelings of Worry, Nervousness, Apprehension or Fear.*

Depression: *A mood disorder that causes a persistent feeling of sadness and loss of interest.*

Administration of magnesium is able to help improve adrenal gland function and it has been shown to be a relaxant of the central nervous system. In many situations it has been used intravenously as a sedative in patients that are unable to relax prior to going into surgery for a procedure.

When you are under serious stress or can't relax, then magnesium can be very beneficial.

Mental and physical stress that is accompanied by a continuous supply of adrenaline will use up magnesium very quickly. Adrenaline is used to affect the heart rate, blood pressure, vascular constriction and muscle contraction and all of these particular actions are dependent upon a sufficient supply of magnesium.

If you have adrenal fatigue it is very important that you don't go too heavy on the magnesium to start with. You may wind up feeling worse than when you started. If you are severely adrenally fatigued, you might be so weak that revving up so many enzyme systems at once can leave you feeling very jittery.

This may make you believe that magnesium is not good for you. However, it is the complete opposite. You could be needing it more than most. Just start with a quarter of the normal dose and work up as your body adjusts.

Studies have also shown that a magnesium deficiency increases anxiety and depression due to the fact that the neurotransmitter required for the brain to feel good (serotonin) depends on magnesium for its production and function.

Research Study #3 - Magnesium and Depression

Yary T et al, "Dietary Intake of Magnesium May Modulate Depression", Biological Trace Element Research, 2013.

This study took 402 postgraduate students in Malaysia and studied them to assess the relationship between magnesium and depressive symptoms. What they found was that magnesium levels were inversely related to depressive symptoms and improved, even after other factors were taken into account, such as sex, age, body mass index, lifestyle and much more…

Research Study #4 – Magnesium and Depression

Tarleton E et al, "The Association between Serum Magnesium Levels and Depression in Adult Primary Care Population", Nutrients, 2019.

In this study, they set out to discover the relationship between serum magnesium and the Patient Health Questionnaire (PHQ – a measure of depression scores).

They analysed 3604 records (mean age 62 years, 42% men) seen in primary care clinics between 2015 and 2018.

The relationship between serum magnesium and deficiency showed a significant effect and for adults seen in primary care, lower serum magnesium levels are associated with depressive symptoms.

Research Study #5 – Magnesium and Anxiety

Boyle N et al, "The effects of Magnesium Supplementation on Subjective Anxiety and Stress – A Systematic Review." Nutrients, 2017.

In this review they set out to determine if magnesium is beneficial for anxiety. Existing evidence is suggestive of a beneficial effect of magnesium on subjective anxiety, although further research needs to be implemented.

Chapter 5 – Arthritis

****

Inflammation of one or more of your joints which causes serious joint pain and stiffness that worsens with age. There are two types of arthritis - osteoarthritis (non-autoimmune) and rheumatoid arthritis (autoimmune). Osteoarthritis most commonly affects the weight bearing joints of the body such as the knees and hips. Women are also much more likely to get it than men, especially after age 50.

It is well known that calcium is needed for bone health and we all know that healthy bones means no arthritis.

As Magnesium deficiency disables the hormone calcitonin, it ends up resulting in calcium being deposited in soft tissue and not into your bones. Therefore, studies recommend decreasing calcium supplementation and/or foods containing a lot of calcium and supplementing with at least 600mg of magnesium per day (it has been shown this can improve arthritis in only 9 months).

However, on top of calcium you need magnesium, boron and vitamin D so as to get maximum calcium absorption.

On top of that, studies have shown that 400-600 IU of Vitamin E can be helpful in the treatment of osteoarthritis.

Research Study #6 - Magnesium and Osteoarthritis

Lee CH et al, "Intra-articular magnesium sulfate (MgSO4) reduces experimental osteoarthritis and nociception: association with attenuation of N-methyl aspartate (NMDA) receptor subunit 1 phosphorylation and apoptosis in chondrocytes", Osteoarthritis Cartilage, 2009

In this animal study, they studied the effects of intra-articular injection of magnesium sulfate and the development of osteoarthritis and to examine the behavioural changes in these animal models. * This study concluded that after receiving the magnesium injections, the animals showed a significantly lower degree of cartilage degeneration than those that didn't receive the injections. Magnesium sulfate also decreased synovitis (inflammation of the synovial membrane).

Chapter 6 - Asthma

****

A respiratory condition which is marked by spasms in the lungs, causing an inability to breathe properly.

Magnesium supplementation has been shown to be beneficial for asthma by reducing the bronchoconstriction and therefore relaxing the muscle around the bronchial tubes. Intravenous solutions of magnesium have often been given to break acute asthma attacks (alongside other nutrients).

As it is a calcium antagonist, it relaxes the airways and smooth muscles and dilates the lungs. It also reduces airway inflammation, inhibits chemicals that initiate spasms and even increases the anti-inflammatory nitric oxide.

Research Study #7 - Magnesium and Lung Function

Britton J et al, "Dietary Magnesium, Lung Function, Wheezing and Airway Hyperactivity In a Random Adult Population Sample", Lancet, 1994.

In this study, 2633 adults aged between 18 and 70 and it was shown that a lower dietary magnesium intake was associated with lower lung function, bronchial hyperactivity and an increased risk of wheezing. The authors of this study concluded that a magnesium deficiency may contribute to the development of asthma and chronic obstructive airway disease.

In this study the subjects were consuming between 600 and 650mg of magnesium per day, taking into account both dietary and supplementary.

Research Study #8 - Magnesium and Asthma

Kazaks AG et al, "Effect of Oral Magnesium Supplementation on measures of airway resistance and subjective assessment of asthma control and quality of life in men and women with mild to moderate asthma: a randomized placebo controlled trial", Journal of Asthma, 2010.

In this study, 55 men and women between the ages of 21 and 55 with mild to moderate asthma were recruited for a 6-month period. These people were split into two groups. The first one received 340mg magnesium per day of magnesium citrate and the other was purely a placebo group.

In this study those who took the magnesium had less reactive airways and a greater predicted improvement over time than those that didn't take the magnesium, therefore confirming that magnesium can in fact relax the bronchial airways and reduce the asthma attacks.

Research Study #9 – Magnesium and Asthma

Skobeloff et al, "Intravenous Magnesium Sulfate for the Treatment of Acute Asthma in the Emergency Department", JAMA, 1989.

Thirty-eight patients suffering from acute exacerbations of moderate to severe asthma were treated in an emergency department with an intravenous infusion of saline placebo or 1.2g of magnesium sulfate after conventional beta-agonist therapy failed to produce significant improvement in peak expiratory flow rate.

Nineteen patients were randomized into each of two groups in a placebo-controlled double-blind clinical trial.

The treatment group demonstrated an increase in peak expiratory flow rate from 225 to 297 L/min as compared with 208 to 216 L/min seen in the placebo group.

In addition, the number admitted via discharged was significantly better for the treatment group (7 vs 12) than the placebo group (15 v 4).

Intravenous magnesium sulfate may represent a beneficial adjunct therapy in patients with moderate to severe asthma who show little improvement with beta-agonists.

Chapter 7 - Autism

****

This condition is defined as a mental condition that is present from early childhood and is characterized by a difficulty in communicating with others and in using language and abstract concepts.

Studies have shown that people with autism suffer from leaky gut syndrome, which means they are not absorbing the necessary minerals even when they are present in the gut. As magnesium absorption is absolutely reliant on intestinal health, a serious magnesium deficiency can occur in adults and children with autism.

If the gut is not healed prior to taking magnesium supplementation, it does not matter how much magnesium is taken because it will not be absorbed.

A combination of Vitamin B6 and Magnesium benefits nearly 50% of all children with the autism spectrum disorder and it has been shown that after two months of treatment, the childrens social, communicative, behavioral and function systems reduced. That is, until the treatment was discontinued and the symptoms returned.

Research Study #10 – Magnesium and Hyperexcitability

Mousain-Bosc et al, "Magnesium Vitamin B6 Intake reduces central nervous system hyperexcitability in children", Journal of the American College of Nutrition, 2004.

This study measured the effects of Magnesium/Vitamin B6 regimen on the behavior of 52 children that were hyper-excitable. So that they were able to measure the magnesium within the cells, they measured the intra erythrocyte levels (ERC).

In 30 of these 52 children they had low ERC levels. Combined Magnesium and Vitamin B6 supplementation of 100mg/day for 3 to 24 weeks restored the levels of magnesium within the cells. In all of the patients, symptoms of excitability, such as physical aggressivity, instability, short attention span etc were reduced after only 1-6 months of treatment.

Therefore, they concluded that even though hyper-excitable children with low intracellular magnesium levels and normal serum levels, supplementing with magnesium can improve this abnormal behaviour.

Chapter 8 - Autoimmune Disorders

****

An autoimmune condition is one where the body's own immune system has gone wrong and starts to attack healthy tissue. For instance, Hashimotos is when the immune system is attacking the thyroid gland and Rheumatoid Arthritis is when the immune system is attacking the joints.

Unfortunately, there has not been a lot of research done on how magnesium affects autoimmune disease as a whole but there have been some studies done independently on certain autoimmune conditions such as Lupus and Rheumatoid Arthritis.

The major reason that magnesium can help with autoimmune conditions is that it is beneficial in reducing inflammation.

There are a couple of other supplements that are beneficial for those with an autoimmune condition, such as:

- Zinc - People with autoimmune disease generally test low in zinc;

- Selenium - This is a powerful antioxidant and is very important for autoimmunity (possibly the most important).

The topic of autoimmunity is such a massive topic that I can't go into great detail in this book but there are many other great resources out there that go into this topic in much greater detail.

Research Study #11 – Magnesium and Systemic Lupus Erythematosus (SLE)

Romano TJ, "Magnesium Deficiency In Systemic Lupus Erythematosus", Journal of Nutritional and Environmental Medicine, 1997

In this study, which was intended to figure out if hypomagnemesia had an effect on SLE patients, red blood cell and plasma magnesium levels were measured. This study measured magnesium levels in SLE, Fibromyalgia and other pain disorders.

What they found was that magnesium levels were lower in people with significant chronic pain and as so many people with autoimmune conditions are in constant pain in stands to reason that magnesium could be beneficial.

Research Study #12 – Magnesium and Hashimoto's Thyroiditis

Kunling W et al, "Severely low serum magnesium is associated with increased risks of positive anti-thyroglobulin antibody and hypo-thyroidism : A Cross Sectional Study", Scientific Reports, 2018.

In this study, they investigated the relationship between low serum magnesium, autoimmune thyroiditis, and thyroid function in 1,257 Chinese Participants.

Demographic data was collected via questionnaires and levels of serum thyroid stimulating hormone, anti-thyroid peroxidase antibody, anti-thyroglobulin antibody (TGAb), free thyroxine, serum magnesium, serum iodine, and urinary iodine concentration was measured.

The risks of TGAb positivity and Hashimoto's Thyroiditis (HT) diagnosed using ultrasonography in the lowest quartile group were higher than those in the adequate magnesium group. Severely low serum magnesium levels are associated with an increased rate of TGAb positivity, HT and Hypothyroidism.

Research Study #13 – Magnesium and Autoimmune Arthritis

Brenner et al, "Short-Term Low Magnesium Diet reduces Autoimmune Arthritis Severity and Synovial Tissue Gene Expression.", Physiol Genomics, 2017.

In this study, DA rats were put on one of three diet regimens before the induction of autoimmune pristine-induced arthritis. They were placed on a 4-week low magnesium diet (food sources), normal diet and magnesium supplemented diet. After 14 days, these rats were switched to a normal diet.

Arthritis severity was scored for 38 days and joints were examined by histology. They found that the rats on the low magnesium diet were significantly and reproducibly protected with 70% lower median arthritis severity score. However, rats on the normal or magnesium supplemented diets did not have this effect. This study reveals a novel role for dietary magnesium in the regulation of autoimmune arthritis and opens new possibilities for the treatment of autoimmune diseases such as Rheumatoid Arthritis and Psoriatic Arthritis with short courses of dietary or drug induced modulation of magnesium levels.

Chapter 9 - Cardiovascular Disease

****

A group of disorders of the heart and blood vessels that include, but are not limited to heart disease, cerebrovascular disease and coronary heart disease.

This vital mineral is absolutely critical to heart health. In order for this muscle to function and orchestrate the very complex process of keeping the heart beating, your magnesium level must be optimal.

While there has been such emphasis on LDL cholesterol, HDL cholesterol, high blood pressure and metabolic syndrome as the cause of heart disease, many studies have indicated that we may actually be looking at the wrong factors. Studies have actually shown that magnesium deficiency may actually be the major contributing factor towards heart disease.

Magnesium allows the arterial muscular tissue to relax and therefore a deficiency can cause the heart to spasm, causing a coronary artery supplying the heart muscle with oxygen to clamp shut without warning. What is interesting to note is that although people think that heart attacks occur because of a build-up of plaque in the coronary arteries, 25% of the heart attacks that occur are actually in people with clean arteries. What's even more disturbing is that numerous studies have shown that a deficiency in magnesium is a contributing factor towards people dying suddenly from ischemic heart disease or other heart related issues.

Magnesium is absolutely critical for the assimilation of calcium. If you have a deficiency in magnesium it can cause a buildup of calcium in the bones and tissues throughout the body. In reference to the heart, if this calcification occurs around the coronary artery, which feeds the heart with the blood and oxygen the result can be sudden death.

Research Study #14 – Magnesium and Cardiovascular Biology

Altura et al, "Magnesium and Cardiovascular Biology: An Important Link between cardiovascular risk factors and atherogenesis", Cellular and Molecular Biology Research, 1995.

In this study it has shown that a reduction in extracellular and intracellular magnesium can cause an entire cascade of pathophysiological issues that promote heart disease.

Research Study #15 – Magnesium and CHD/SCD

Kieboom B et al, "Serum Magnesium and the Risk of Death from Coronary Heart Disease and Sudden Cardiac Death", J Am Heart Association, 2016.

Nine-thousand eight-hundred and twenty participants (mean age 65.1 years, 56.8% female) were included with a median follow-up of 8.7 years.

They found that a very small increase in serum magnesium level was associated with a lower risk for CHD mortality. Low serum magnesium was associated with an increased risk of CHD mortality and SCD, as well as accelerated subclinical atherosclerosis.

Low magnesium was associated with both carotid intima-media thickness and heart rate. Further research required.

Research Study #16 – Magnesium and Cardiovascular Heart Failure

Ceremuzynski L et al, "Hypomagnesemia in Heart Failure with Ventricular Arrhythmias. Beneficial effects of Magnesium Supplementation.", J Intern Med, 2000.

A total of 78 patients entered and 68 patients completed the study.

Serum magnesium and potassium levels, urine magnesium excretion and the incidence of ventricular arrhythmias were assessed throughout the study.

The patients who displayed complex arrhythmias after the first week of hospital medication were randomised 2:1 to double-blind magnesium supplementation or placebo.

Intravenous administration of magnesium (magnesium sulphate 8g in 250mL of 5% glucose) or placebo (250 mL of 5% glucose) over 12 hours.

Hypomagnesemia, probably related to increased urine magnesium excretion, is an essential feature of heart failure associated with complex ventricular arrhythmias. These arrhythmias can be alleviated/abolished by magnesium supplementation.

Chapter 10 - Cavities

****

A decayed part of a tooth.

I bet you are probably curious as to how magnesium can help with dental health. For years we have been told that we have to increase our calcium and more recently our Vitamin D levels to protect our teeth from cavities and other dental issues.

However, what we are often not told is that increasing your magnesium is as important, if not more important than your calcium and vitamin D, because magnesium deficiency is a lot more common than calcium deficiency.

Studies have shown that when calcium and magnesium levels are not in the correct ratio (2:1) there is an increased incidence of periodontal disease. When your calcium and phosphorus levels are in excess, you shut down magnesium's ability to activate thyrocalcitonin which is a hormone that sends calcium to your bones.

What's even more interesting is the latest research showing that poor dental health due to inflammation is a contributor towards heart disease and diabetes and therefore as magnesium lowers inflammation in the body, it also decreases the risk of these conditions.

Numerous studies have shown that it is actually dietary magnesium and not calcium (and definitely not fluoride) that creates glossy, hard, tooth enamel that resists decay and strong and resilient bones.

Chapter 11 - Chronic Fatigue Syndrome

****

This is a condition that has an unknown cause but does consist of a variety of symptoms including fever, aching, prolonged tiredness and depression.

If you are suffering from persistent fatigue that is not due to exertion and is not significantly relieved by rest, and it is not caused by other medical conditions, it is possible that you could be suffering from CFS.

The symptoms of Chronic Fatigue Syndrome can include, but are not limited to:

• Fatigue after exertion;
• Unrefreshing sleep;
• Widespread muscle and joint pain;
• Sore throats;
• Headaches;
• Chronic and severe mental and physical exhaustion; and
• Much More...

Although this condition is relatively rare with only 3000 pieces in every 100,000. It occurs more often in women than men and is very rare in children and adolescents.

However, the good news is that there are supplements that can be taken to help treat chronic fatigue syndrome, of which one of them is magnesium (see studies below).

On top of magnesium there are other supplements that can also be beneficial:

• Essential Fatty Acids - may help reduce fatigue at 1000mg x 3 times per day;

• Vitamin B12 - Injections of B12 at 2500 - 5000 mcg every 2-3 days for several weeks has been shown to improve energy;

• L-Carnitine - 500 - 1000mg x 3 times per day for 8 weeks to support energy

   Herbs such as Ginseng and Echinacea, as well as Homeopathics such as Arsenicum, Gelsemium, Pulsatilla and Sulphur have also been found to help improve Chronic Fatigue Syndromes.

Research Study #17 – Magnesium and Chronic Fatigue Syndrome

IM Cox et al, "Red Blood Cell Magnesium and Chronic Fatigue Syndrome", The Lancet, 1991.

In 1991 a study was done on 32 patients with CFS. When tested all of these patients had reduced levels of serum magnesium. When serum magnesium is very low it is even more concerning due to the fact that the majority of magnesium is found in the tissues and not in the blood. So, if serum magnesium is low, then you know that you are deficient.

Anyway, in this study, 15 of these patients received intramuscular injections of magnesium sulphate every week for 6 weeks and 17 received a placebo. Of the 15 patients that received the magnesium, 12 of them showed an improvement in symptoms, including improved energy, better emotional state and less pain.

Red cell magnesium returned to normal in all patients on magnesium but only in 1 patient on placebo, and as only 3 out of the 17 people on placebo said they felt better it indicates that magnesium plays a role in helping chronic fatigue syndrome.

Research Study #18 – Magnesium and Chronic Fatigue Syndrome

Chilton S.A, "Cognitive Behavior Therapy for the Chronic Fatigue Syndrome. Evening Primrose Oil and Magnesium have been shown to be effective", BMJ, 1996.

In this study, they found that Intramuscular Magnesium Supplements have been given to patients with low red blood cell magnesium in a double-blind controlled placebo trial.

They found that Myalgia and Fatigue improved in about 70% of subjects.

Chapter 12 - Constipation

****

Difficulty emptying the bowels.

Although there is very little research done on the effectiveness of magnesium on constipation, it is still used as a laxative by many.

Magnesium increases water in your intestines which helps to initiate peristalsis, which also helps push food into your stomach. It also helps to relax the muscles in your intestines and attracts water which softens the stools, making it easier to pass.

As the intestines will be absorbing a lot of this water, it is very important that you drink a lot of water after taking magnesium.

Another factor that you need to take into consideration is whether or not you are taking calcium supplements. Calcium is known to constipate you (especially if it is calcium carbonate) and therefore if you do take these supplements, try switching to calcium citrate and make sure you are also taking magnesium supplementation.

On top of magnesium, Black Psyllium has been found to also be effective at treating constipation.

Research Study #19 – Magnesium and Constipation

Murakami K et al, "Association between Dietary Fiber, Water and Magnesium Intake and functional constipation amongst Japanese women", European Journal of Clinical Nutrition, 2006.

In this study, it consisted of 3835 Japanese women, with a prevalence of functional constipation of 26.2%. They found that neither dietary fibre OR water from fluids were associated with constipation. Instead, they found that low intakes of water from foods, as well as low magnesium levels are associated with an increased risk of functional constipation.

Chapter 13 - Diabetes/Insulin Resistance

****

Insulin Resistance is when the cells fail to respond to normal actions of insulin. Although the pancreas still produces insulin, the cells do not hear the call and therefore have to keep pumping out more and more insulin. This leads to high blood sugar levels and eventually Type II Diabetes.

Magnesium supplementation has been found to be beneficial in improving insulin sensitivity and clinicians have even gone so far as to say that they believe replenishing the body of magnesium can help to delay Type 2 Diabetes, as well as warding off its complications, such as cardiovascular disease, retinopathy and nephropathy.

Research has shown that diabetics - both Type 1 and Type 2 generally have lower plasma magnesium levels than those without diabetes. What's even more important to test is the intracellular free magnesium levels in the erythrocytes. This level has been shown to also be lower in patients with Type 2 Diabetes.

Both extracellular and intracellular magnesium deficiency has been found in chronic Type 2 Diabetics, which could put them at a much greater risk of cardiovascular disease. Studies have also shown that lower serum levels of magnesium increase the likelihood or progression of retinopathy in both Type 1 and Type 2 Diabetics. Insulin Resistance, which is also a side effect of Diabetes actually causes reduced intracellular magnesium and therefore by giving additional magnesium it can ward off that insulin resistance.

So, why is it that Diabetics tend to suffer from a magnesium deficiency? Studies have shown, there are really 4 reasons why this may be occurring:

- Their diets tend to be low in magnesium;
- Their excretion of magnesium from the urine seems to be a lot higher;
- Insulin Resistance affects magnesium transport and glucose metabolism; and
- If you are taking Diuretics, it could promote muscle wasting.

Summary - Adding magnesium supplementation can not only help with the insulin resistance associated with Diabetes, but also decreases the risk of becoming afflicted with Type 2 Diabetes to start with, and all of its associated complications...

Chapter 14 - Dysmenorrhea

****

Painful menstruation, typically involving abdominal cramps.

When it comes to dysmenorrhea, there are two different types that we need to consider:

Primary

Usually starts within several years after your first menstrual period, which involves no physical abnormality. Hormone substances such as prostaglandins are produced naturally in the body and are thought to be a cause of the menstrual cramps, pain and inflammation.

Secondary

This is when there the painful periods are caused by another condition, such as endometriosis, pelvic inflammatory disease, uterine fibroids or uterine polyps.

Studies have shown that magnesium is very effective at reducing the pain and much less additional pain killers were required.

On top of magnesium, there are other supplements and techniques that have been shown to be useful for helping to alleviate dysmenorrhea:

- Vitamin B1;
- Fish Oils;
- Acupressure;
- Calcium;
- Fennel;
- Crampbark;
- Acupressure;
- Heat;
- Exercise.

Research Study #20 – Magnesium and Dysmenorrhea

Fontana-Kleiber H, "Therapeutic Effects of Magnesium in Dysmenorrhea", Clinical Trial, 1990.

In this study, the therapeutic effect of magnesium was investigated in 32 women (16 to 42 years old) who have been treated for primary dysmenorrhea. At the end of the study (6 cycles) they were able to analyse the results in 21 patients, 11 in magnesium group and 10 in placebo.

What they found was that even in the magnesium group, pain was still felt but in the second and third day, the magnesium group experienced less back pain and lower abdominal pain than those in the placebo group. There was also a marked decrease in absences from work due to dysmenorrhea in those taking magnesium.

Research Study #21 – Magnesium and Dysmenorrhea

Parazzini et al, "Magnesium in the Gynecological Practice: A Literature Review", Magnes Res, 2017

In this review, they pointed out that there is a growing amount of evidence suggesting that magnesium deficiency may play an important role in several female conditions such as PMS, Dysmenorrhea and Postmenopausal Symptoms.

It highlighted that there seems to be a positive correlation between magnesium administration and relief or prevention of the symptoms, therefore suggesting magnesium may be a viable solution for these conditions.

Research Study #22 – Magnesium and Dysmenorrhea

Fontana-Klaiber et al, "Therapeutic Effects of Magnesium in Dysmenorrhea", Schweiz Rundsch Med Prax, 1990

In a randomized double-blind study, the therapeutic effect of magnesium was investigated in 32 women (of which 21 completed). The women were split up into 2 groups – 11 taking magnesium and 10 that were placebo. The magnesium group showed a therapeutic effect on back pain and lower abdominal pain on the second and third day of the cycle. There was also reduced numbers of absences from work due to it.

Magnificent Magnesium

Chapter 15 - Fibromyalgia

****

A rheumatic condition which is characterized by muscular/musculoskeletal pain with stiffness and localized tenderness at specific points on the body.

Fibromyalgia is a condition that has caused confusion amongst the medical community for years, at least that was until recently. New research has shown that fibromyalgia is actually a disorder associated with a heightened sense of pain. So basically, sensations which should normally be interpreted by the brain as being non-painful can be extremely painful with Fibromyalgia.

In fact, I was consulting with one client in the clinic who had fibromyalgia. She suffered from intense pain on a daily basis and after she came in, I told her I would give her a remedial massage one day. I had barely touched her skin when she almost jumped off the table, screaming in pain.

When you are magnesium deficient it often causes a constant state of muscular spasms, therefore contributing to the constant pains experienced by fibromyalgia sufferers.

Aside from magnesium there is one other supplement that is seen as incredibly useful when it comes to fibromyalgia and that is Malic Acid. This is another supplement that has shown improvement in pain within 48 hours of supplementing with 1200-2400mg of Malic Acid.

Research Study #23 – Magnesium and Fibromyalgia

Selda Bagis et al, *"Is Magnesium Citrate treatment effective on pain, clinical parameters and functional status in people with fibromyalgia"*, Rheumatology International, 2012.

60 women who were diagnosed with fibromyalgia and 20 women without (of the same age group) were assessed for pain intensity, pain threshold, number of tender points and other parameters. Serum magnesium levels and intracellular magnesium levels were tested. Consisted of 3 groups: Mag Citrate (300mg/day), Amitryptiline (antidepressant) and Combination Mag Citrate and Amitryptiline.

They found those with fibromyalgia had lower magnesium levels than those in the healthy group. All parameters decreased in Magnesium Group and Combined Group.

Chapter 16 - Hypercholesterolemia

****

An excess of cholesterol in the bloodstream.

Cholesterol has been given far too much credit when it comes to heart disease. The overuse of statin drugs is extremely concerning, considering the dangerous side effects of it and considering how easy it is to really maximize your cholesterol for optimal health. You will notice I didn't say to lower your cholesterol because the story is a lot more complex than that.

For instance, studies have actually shown that cholesterol is protective, especially when talking about HDL levels. Even LDL is not as bad as it seems as long as it is the right type - the big fluffy kind instead of the small dense particles. What you have to really look out for are triglycerides which are primarily caused by excess consumption of carbohydrates.

Cholesterol is absolutely critical for optimal cell health and is a building block for essential hormones, such as testosterone and estrogen etc. So what do you think happens if you reduce your cholesterol too low. You do not have a sufficient supply to produce the hormones you need, and as hormones pretty much run our bodies, that is not a good thing.

What's even more, statins have never been proven to be effective with anyone and especially not women. Not only study has been done at this point in time showing that statins are effective at preventing heart disease in women and the only studies done have been in middle aged men, and even then, the results are dismal.

However, what is rather disturbing is the fact that websites out there are still claiming how effective they are. Plus, they have as a warning sign on the box: This product may cause memory loss, mental confusion, high blood sugar and type 2 diabetes. Not exactly an advertisement for taking them is it.

Anyway, I guess that is enough for right now about cholesterol and statins. The use of statin drugs really concerns me, especially because my mum was taking them with very serious side effects and definitely no help whatsoever. She trusted what the doctors told her, especially as they scared her into taking them.

But maybe if you are on statin drugs you are asking the question right now: But they are bringing my cholesterol down, isn't that good? My answer to that is "not necessarily". Studies have shown that people with higher cholesterol levels live longer than those with low cholesterol. Isn't that surprising?

OK, on to how magnesium actually helps with high cholesterol levels. This can be a little tricky to understand with biochemical pathways and such, but I will try to make it as easy to understand as possible.

Studies have found that one of the top items on the list of things you can use to reduce the bad LDL cholesterol (small, dense particles), reduce triglycerides and increase HDL cholesterol is magnesium. Magnesium acts like a natural statin drug but without the harmful side effects of muscle pain and joint pain etc. However, statin drugs only decrease the LDL cholesterol, they do not reduce triglycerides and they have very minimal effect on increasing HDL levels.

Now to the scientific part. In order for the body to make cholesterol it requires an enzyme called HMG-CoA reductase. This enzyme is the one that makes sure there is only enough cholesterol in its body as is needed, and therefore stops cholesterol from being overproduced and deposited in places it shouldn't be deposited. Well, magnesium is required for that enzyme to be regulated.

This enzyme is the same enzyme that is regulated by statins, except that statins destroy the mechanism altogether causing a lot more issues in the body.

Research Study #24 – Magnesium and Cholesterol

Olatunji LA et al, "Effect of Increased Magnesium Intake On Plasma Cholesterol, Triglycerides and Oxidative Stress in alloxan-diabetic rats", African Journal of Medical Sciences, 2007

In this study they found that diets rich in magnesium could exert cardioprotective effects through reducing plasma total cholesterol, triglyceride and also ameliorated HDL cholesterol/total cholesterol ratio. The plasma ascorbic acid and magnesium in the rats was also increased.

Now, although this study was done in rats, it does show promise in detailing how magnesium may help the human cohort too.

Chapter 17 – Hypertension (High Blood Pressure)

****

Elevated Blood Pressure.

If you are dealing with hypertension, then magnesium is one supplement that should definitely be integrated into your medicine cabinet.

There have been many studies done highlighting the benefits of using magnesium for the treatment of hypertension, although it does seem to be more effective when the magnesium is obtained from food sources. This could be due to the fact that the food sources will also include the other important electrolytes too.

It is important to note that in order for magnesium to help with blood pressure, you need to first be deficient in it and not getting enough from your diet.

However, if you are deficient, magnesium will help by preventing blood vessels from constricting and increasing blood flow, therefore reducing your blood pressure.

On top of this, magnesium regulates the level of sodium, potassium and calcium within the cells. Sodium and Potassium work together to maintain normal blood pressure levels and needs to be balanced.

Research Study #25 – Magnesium and Hypertension

Zhang X et al, "Effects of Magnesium Supplementation on Blood Pressure", Hypertension, 2016

In this meta-analysis, they aimed to quantify the effect of oral Magnesium Supplementation on blood pressure by synthesizing the evidence from randomized, double blind, placebo-controlled trials.

34 trials involving 2028 participants were eligible for this meta-analysis.

They found that Magnesium Supplementation at a median dose of 368 mg/d for 3 months significantly reduced systolic BP by 2.00 mmHg and diastolic BP by 1.78 mmHg and showed an increase of 0.05 mmol/L of serum magnesium. This shows a causal effect of Mg Supplementation.

Chapter 18 - Kidney Stones

****

A hard mass formed in the kidneys, typically consisting of insoluble calcium compounds.

The prevalence of kidney stones is high amongst those in the 30-45-year old age group and high urinary calcium is often the cause. Once these kidney stones develop the patients will unfortunately have a 50% - 75% chance of developing them again.

It has been shown that people who are magnesium deficient have a much greater chance of suffering from calcium oxalate stones. By increasing calcium solubility, magnesium has been shown to be able to prevent kidney stones, especially in people who suffer from them regularly.

Aside from magnesium, Vitamin B6 is an important nutrient in preventing the formation of kidney stones. It is effective at preventing kidney stones through its effect on oxalate metabolism and as some people produce excess oxalate, B6 is helpful at modulating that.

Ensuring that you are drinking plenty of water is also very important as studies have shown that too little water can encourage the precipitation of calcium into stones and therefore chronic dehydration is one of the primary causes of kidney stones. Plus, avoid drinking caffeine as much as you can because that has also been shown to promote the formation of the stones.

Research Study #26 – Magnesium and Kidney Stones

Prien EL Sr et al, "Magnesium oxide-pyridoxine therapy for recurrent calcium oxalate calculi", Journal of Urology, 1974.

149 patients who suffered from an average of 1.3 kidney stones per year were put on 100mg of magnesium oxide per day, 3 times per day and 10mg of pyridoxine once per day for 4.5-6 years. In this time, stone formation fell by a whopping 92.3%, from an average of 1.3 stones per year to 0.1 stones per year.

Chapter 19 - Liver Disease and Cirrhosis

****

A study published in the "Biological Trace Element Research" journal states that alongside zinc and selenium, magnesium levels are decreased in people with liver cirrhosis.

As the liver cirrhosis advances, the deficiency in these trace minerals decrease even further.

Other supplements that have been considered advantageous to healing cirrhosis are:

- Milk Thistle;
- Licorice Root (do not take with high blood pressure);
- Cordyceps;
- SAM-e;
- B Vitamins.

Research Study #27 – Magnesium and Liver Cirrhosis

Biswajit Das et al, "Serum magnesium level in patients with liver cirrhosis", International Journal of Biological Medical Research, 2011.

In this study they had 100 subjects, 50 that had alcoholic induced cirrhosis and 50 normal subjects. Serum magnesium levels were measured in both the groups. This study showed that serum magnesium levels were decreases in all cases of liver cirrhosis.

Research Study #28 – Magnesium and Liver Cirrhosis

Vijaylaxmi Nangliya et al, "Study of Trace Elements in Liver Cirrhosis Patients and Their Role in the Prognosis of Disease", 24th Jan 2015.

150 cirrhotic subjects ranging in age from 20-70 years of age were compared against 50 healthy subjects. They were assessed for severity of disease as either mild, moderate and severe. Routine investigations were done and trace elements (copper, magnesium, zinc and selenium) were analysed. Serum levels of copper was increased, while magnesium, zinc and selenium was decreased.

Chapter 20 - Migraines

****

A recurrent throbbing headache that can cause delirium, dizziness, nausea and disturbed vision.

Migraines can be extremely debilitating and I know because I, myself suffer from them at least once a month. Sometimes it gets so bad that I have to ask my husband to take the kids out of the house because even the slightest whisper can make it feel like somebody is putting a knife through your head.

Migraines have been researched a lot in recent years and they have found that migraines are actually hereditary. As both my parents suffer from migraines I was lucky enough to also be afflicted with them. However, in saying that there is a lot you can do to ward off migraines.

It is no doubt that migraines are caused from changes to blood flow in the brain. There are many triggers that contribute to this debilitating condition:
- Stress;
- Low Blood Sugar;
- Lack of Sleep;
- Hormone Imbalance;
- Temperature Changes/Hot Temperatures;
- Bright Lights;
- Loud Noises;
- Strong Odors;
- Exertion; and
- Vitamin and Mineral Deficiencies.

One of the main vitamin deficiencies is that of magnesium. A deficiency in magnesium allows the neurotransmitter serotonin to flow freely, which can cause vascular spasms, which will then reduce blood flow and oxygen to the brain. It also triggers other pain producing prostaglandins and neuropeptide P.

Many studies show that approximately 50% of migraine sufferers have low magnesium when an attack occurs. Therefore, if you suffer from a migraine how about trying an infusion of magnesium and see if it puts a stop to your migraine. Then, if you ensure you take regular magnesium supplementation you may prevent yourself from getting the attacks to start with.

Research Study #29 – Magnesium and Migraines

Koseoglu, E et al, "The effects of magnesium prophylaxi in migraine without aura", Magnesium Research, 2008

In this study, they took 30 patients with a migraine with an aura, and 10 patients with similar conditions in the other group. The 30 patients in group 1 were taking magnesium while the 10 in the other group were not. Migraine attack severity and frequency were recorded, and they found this severity and frequency was diminished in those with magnesium.

This indicates that magnesium is a beneficial agent in prophylaxis of migraine without aura and it may work with both vascular and neurogenic mechanisms.

Research Study #30 – Magnesium and All Headache Types

Mauskop A et al, "Intravenous Magnesium Sulphate Rapidly Alleviates Headaches of Various Types", Headache, 1996.

This study set out to evaluate the efficacy of an intravenous infusion of 1g magnesium sulfate for the treatment of patients with headaches. They also determined whether patients with certain headache types exhibit low serum magnesium as opposed to total serum magnesium.

This study consisted of 40 patients: 16 with migraines without aura, 9 with clustr headaches, 4 with chronic tension-type headaches and 11 with chronic migrainous headaches. Complete elimination of pain was observed in 80% of the patients within 15 minutes of the infusion. In 56% of the patients, there was no recurrence or worsening of pain within 24 hours. In 18 of the patients, the pain relief lasted for at least 24 hours and 16 of them had low serum magnesium levels. Those who did not have pain return had the lowest magnesium levels, while those non-responders had the highest levels.

They also found that those with cluster headaches typically had the lowest basal levels of magnesium, while all types except for chronic tension had high Calcium to Magnesium Ratio's. Low serum and brain tissue ionized magnesium levels may precipitate headache symptoms in susceptible people.

Chapter 21 - Osteoporosis

****

A medical condition where the bones become brittle and fragile from loss of tissue, typically caused by changes in hormones and deficiencies in numerous vitamins/minerals.

It is a well-known fact that calcium is an important mineral for the bones but what most people don't know is that without magnesium, you could actually be causing bone loss as opposed to bone growth.

Magnesium is important for working with the thyroid and parathyroid glands to support bone health. It does this by stimulating the production of calcitonin, a bone preserving hormone and it also regulates parathyroid hormone, which regulates bone breakdown in a number of ways.

Magnesium is also necessary for conversion of Vitamin D to its active form. Vitamin D is another nutrient that is required for optimal bone health. A deficiency in magnesium can result in Vitamin D resistance.

Studies have shown that low magnesium intake, as well as low blood and bone magnesium levels is widely associated with osteoporosis in women.

Research Study #31 – Magnesium and Osteoporosis

JE Sojka, "Magnesium Supplementation and Osteoporosis", Nutrition Reviews, 1995.

In this study, a group of menopausal women were given magnesium hydroxide to assess the effects of magnesium on bone density.

They found that after 2 years, the magnesium appeared to prevent fractures and result in an increase in bone density.

Chapter 22 - PMS

****

Magnesium supplementation has been found to be very useful when it comes to treating premenstrual syndrome and common symptoms such as cramping, irritability, fatigue, breast tenderness, depression and water retention are alleviated.

It is important to note that magnesium is at its lowest during menstruation, and therefore supplementation can relieve these symptoms. Supplementation of at least 500mg-1000mg per day are currently recommended for those with PMS.

On top of magnesium, there are a number of other supplements that are useful for helping to treat PMS, of which some are:

• Calcium Citrate - 500-1000mg per day may help reduce PMS symptoms;

• Vitamin D - alongside the vitamin D, take at least 400IU daily so as to help with PMS;

• Omega 3 Fatty Acids - reduces inflammation;

• Evening Primrose Oil - 500-1000mg per day is a great source of gamma linoleic acid and is very effective at treating PMS.

Research Study #32 – Magnesium and PMS

Quaranta S, "Pilot Study of the efficacy and safety of a modified-release magnesium mg tablet for the treatment of premenstrual syndrome", Clinical Drug Investigation, 2007.

Several studies have reported lower intracellular magnesium concentrations in people with PMS. This study assessed the efficacy and safety of a modified magnesium tablet for improving symptoms of PMS in women.

After a 3-month observational period of women between the ages of 18 and 45 years with a regular menstrual cycle that have been affected by PMS, the modified release tablets were given to each of these women over 3 menstrual cycles.What they found was that PMS symptoms significantly improved in those people taking magnesium.

Chapter *23 - Restless Leg Syndrome*

****

This is an extremely uncomfortable condition that causes a strong urge to move your legs. These sensations can feel tingly, prickly or even like you have small insects crawling all over you.

Various studies have shown that magnesium can be extremely beneficial for Restless Leg Syndrome and in actual fact some have even speculated that it is caused by a magnesium deficiency.

Magnesium is important for relaxing the nerves and preventing calcium from rushing into the nerve cells to activate them. However, in the case of a magnesium deficiency the nerve cells can become overactive and send too many messages to the muscles, causing the muscles to constantly contract.

Research Study #33 – Magnesium and Restless Leg Syndrome

Hornyak M et al, "Magnesium Therapy for periodic leg movements-related insomnia and restless leg syndrome: an open pilot study", Sleep, 1998.

In this study, observations have shown that oral magnesium therapy may ameliorate symptoms in people with moderate restless leg syndrome. A dose of 12.4 mmol of magnesium was administered in the evening over a period of 4-6 weeks. They found that magnesium improved sleep efficiency and reduced sleep arousal time. Therefore, this study concluded that magnesium treatment may be a useful alternative therapy in patients with mild or moderate Restless Leg Syndrome related insomnia.

Research Study #34 – Magnesium and Periodic Leg Movement

Marshall N et al, "Magnesium Supplementation for the Treatment of Restless Leg Syndrome and Periodic Limb Movement Disorder: A Systematic Review.

This study found that after magnesium was administered orally, the periodic leg movements with arousal decreased significantly and that without arousal also decreased moderately. It also improved sleep efficiency.

Chapter 24 - Thyroid Disorders

****

Hypothyroidism is an abnormally low activity of the thyroid gland which can result in problems with growth and mental development in both children and adults.

Hyperthyroidism is an overactivity of the thyroid gland, resulting in a rapid heartbeat and an increased rate of metabolism.

Hypothyroidism

One of the biggest problems associated with a magnesium deficiency is that of thyroid issues. Hypothyroidism (low thyroid function) can make it hard for your body to lose weight or keep off excess weight. A lack of magnesium does not directly cause hypothyroidism but it does impact the thyroid in a round-about way.

It synergizes the function of the parathyroid gland which regulates vitamin c and magnesium absorption.

Hyperthyroidism

Studies have shown that the excessive production of thyroid hormone decreases the absorption of magnesium, therefore making a deficiency of this mineral likely. They have also shown that some people with hyperthyroidism and graves disease (autoimmune condition of the thyroid gland) notice a significant decrease in their heart palpitations when they supplement with magnesium.

Research Study #35 – Magnesium and Thyroid

Abdel Gayoum AA, "Dyslipidemia and serum mineral profiles in patients with thyroid disorders", Saudi Medical Journal, 2014.

The purpose of this study was to investigate changes in serum lipid profiles, level of serum minerals associated with thyroid disorders and compare these with the serum lipid and mineral profiles in hypothyroid patients receiving thyroxine.

They found that hypothyroidism caused impaired renal function, glucose intolerance, hyperlipidemia and a reduction in serum phosphates. Hyperthyroidism on the hand caused a reduction in serum lipids, magnesium and potassium.

****

SECTION 3 – FINAL WORDS...

****

Chapter #24 – Summary Checklist

****

1. Incorporate as many magnesium rich foods as possible;

2. Ensure you get adequate sleep every night. If you are having trouble sleeping, take some magnesium prior to sleeping;

3. Reduce your alcohol consumption;

4. Reduce your coffee consumption;

5. If you have mercury fillings, consider seeing a holistic dentist and get them removed as soon as possible because mercury is known to inhibit absorption of magnesium;

6. Reduce or Eliminate Soft Drinks completely as the phosphoric acid inhibits absorption;

7. If you are on birth control pills at all ensure that you take a magnesium supplement;

8. If you come into contact with fluoride, through non-filtered water, showers or toothpaste, make sure you take magnesium so that it offsets the negative effects of the fluoride;

9. Heal Your Gut from any possibly Leaky Gut Syndrome you may be experiencing;

10. Manage your stress levels as much as possible as stress depletes your body of magnesium.

Conclusion

****

So, firstly I want to thank you for reading through to the end of the book. I am hoping by now that you are convinced how important magnesium is for optimal health and with it being completely safe in most cases, it may be something you could find useful in implementing.

If you are suffering from any of the conditions listed or you are lacking in energy and would just like to feel better, then seriously consider giving magnesium a go.

I consider magnesium to be my drug of choice and if I was giving a choice of 3 supplements to recommend, this would definitely be at the top of my list.

3 Places You Can Get Magnesium...

Option #1 - Worldwide

No matter where you are, a good option for finding some suitable magnesium is finding a local health food store and seeing what magnesium they have on offer. Remember to take my book with you if possible so you can see what the best types of magnesium are for you.

Option #2 - Most countries (some only available in US) - Amazon via my store

I have sourced out some magnesium products that I believe are of great quality. If you would like to check this out, you can go to http://www.asknaturopathjen.com/store

Option #3 - Australia Only

If you live in Australia, you are able to contact me via email at jen@asknaturopathjen.com and let me know what you are requiring. I have suppliers where I can get some good quality supplements and I can have them shipped to you anywhere in Australia.

Testimonials

****

So, what are you waiting for? Get yourself some magnesium and see how great you can feel. Once you have tried it please email me at jen@asknaturopathjen.com and give me a testimonial on how magnesium has helped you. This would be awesome!!!

Once again, thanks very much for reading my book. If you would like to check out the references associated with this book, please see below. I have spent a lot of time and effort researching all the information I have given, and I hope it has given you some insight into the amazing wonders of "Magnificent Magnesium".

****

SECTION 4 – REFERENCES

****

Scientific References

****

1.   Starobrat-Hermelin B et al, *"The effects of Magnesium Physiological Supplementation on Hyperactivity in Children with Attention Deficit Hyperactivity Disorder (ADHD). Positive Response to Magnesium Oral Loading Test"*, Magnesium Research, 1997

2.   Hemamy M et al, *"Effect of Vitamin D and Magnesium Supplementation on Behavior Problems in Children with Attention-Deficit Hyperactivity Disorder"*, Int J Prev Med, 2020.

3.   Yary T et al, *"Dietary Intake of Magnesium May Modulate Depression"*, Biological Trace Element Research, 2013.

4.   Tarleton E et al, *"The Association between Serum Magnesium Levels and Depression in Adult Primary Care Population"*, Nutrients, 2019.

5.   Boyle N et al, *"The effects of Magnesium Supplementation on Subjective Anxiety and Stress – A Systematic Review"* Nutrients, 2017.

6.   Lee CH et al, *"Intra-articular magnesium sulfate (MgSO4) reduces experimental osteoarthritis and nociception: association with attenuation of N-methyl aspartate (NMDA) receptor subunit 1 phosphorylation and apoptosis in chondrocytes"*, Osteoarthritis Cartilage, 2009

7.   Britton J et al, *"Dietary Magnesium, Lung Function, Wheezing and Airway Hyperactivity in a Random Adult Population Sample"*, Lancet, 1994.

8.   Kazaks AG et al, *"Effect of Oral Magnesium Supplementation on measures of airway resistance and subjective assessment of asthma control and quality of life in men and women with mild to moderate asthma: a randomized placebo-controlled trial"*, Journal of Asthma, 2010.

9.   Skobeloff et al, *"Intravenous Magnesium Sulfate for the Treatment of Acute Asthma in the Emergency Department"*, JAMA, 1989.

10. Mousain-Bosc et al, *"Magnesium Vitamin B6 Intake reduces central nervous system hyperexcitability in children"*, Journal of the American College of Nutrition, 2004.

11. Romano TJ, *"Magnesium Deficiency In Systemic Lupus Erythematosus"*, Journal of Nutritional and Environmental Medicine, 1997.

12. Kunling W et al, *"Severely low serum magnesium is associated with increased risks of positive anti-thyroglobulin antibody and hypothyroidism: A Cross Sectional Study"*, Scientific Reports, 2018.

13. Brenner et al, *"Short-Term Low Magnesium Diet reduces Autoimmune Arthritis Severity and Synovial Tissue Gene Expression"*, Physiol Genomics, 2017.

14. Altura et al, *"Magnesium and Cardiovascular Biology: An Important Link between cardiovascular risk factors and atherogenesis"*, Cellular and Molecular Biology Research, 1995.

15. Kieboom B et al, *"Serum Magnesium and the Risk of Death from Coronary Heart Disease and Sudden Cardiac Death"*, J Am Heart Association, 2016.

16. Ceremuzynski L et al, *"Hypomagnesemia in Heart Failure with Ventricular Arrhythmias. Beneficial effects of Magnesium Supplementation"*, J Intern Med, 2000.

17. IM Cox et al, *"Red Blood Cell Magnesium and Chronic Fatigue Syndrome"*, The Lancet, 1991.

18. Chilton S.A, *"Cognitive Behavior Therapy for the Chronic Fatigue Syndrome. Evening Primrose Oil and Magnesium have been shown to be effective"*, BMJ, 1996.

19. Murakami K et al, *"Association between Dietary Fiber, Water and Magnesium Intake and functional constipation amongst Japanese women"*, European Journal of Clinical Nutrition, 2006.

20. Fontana-Kleiber H, *"Therapeutic Effects of Magnesium in Dysmenorrhea"*, Clinical Trial, 1990.

21. Parazzini et al, *"Magnesium in the Gynecological Practice: A Literature Review"*, Magnes Res, 2017

22. Fontana-Klaiber et al, *"Therapeutic Effects of Magnesium in Dysmenorrhea"*, Schweiz Rundsch Med Prax, 1990

23. Selda Bagis et al, *"Is Magnesium Citrate treatment effective on pain, clinical parameters and functional status in people with fibromyalgia"*, Rheumatology International, 2012.

24. Olatunji LA et al, *"Effect of Increased Magnesium Intake On Plasma Cholesterol, Triglycerides and Oxidative Stress in alloxan-diabetic rats"*, African Journal of Medical Sciences, 2007

25. Zhang X et al, *"Effects of Magnesium Supplementation on Blood Pressure"*, Hypertension, 2016

26. Prien EL Sr et al, *"Magnesium oxide-pyridoxine therapy for recurrent calcium oxalate calculi"*, Journal of Urology, 1974.

27. Biswajit Das et al, *"Serum magnesium level in patients with liver cirrhosis"*, International Journal of Biological Medical Research, 2011.

28. Vijaylaxmi Nangliya et al, *"Study of Trace Elements in Liver Cirrhosis Patients and Their Role in the Prognosis of Disease"*, 24th Jan 2015.

29. Koseoglu, E et al, *"The effects of magnesium prophylaxi in migraine without aura"*, Magnesium Research, 2008

30. Mauskop A et al, *"Intravenous Magnesium Sulphate Rapidly Alleviates Headaches of Various Types"*, Headache, 1996.

31. JE Sojka, *"Magnesium Supplementation and Osteoporosis"*, Nutrition Reviews, 1995.

32. Quaranta S, *"Pilot Study of the efficacy and safety of a modified-release magnesium mg tablet for the treatment of premenstrual syndrome"*, Clinical Drug Investigation, 2007.

33. Hornyak M et al, *"Magnesium Therapy for periodic leg movements-related insomnia and restless leg syndrome: an open pilot study"*, Sleep, 1998.

34. Marshall N et al, *"Magnesium Supplementation for the Treatment of Restless Leg Syndrome and Periodic Limb Movement Disorder: A Systematic Review"*, Sleep Medicine Reviews, 2019

35. Abdel Gayoum AA, *"Dyslipidemia and serum mineral profiles in patients with thyroid disorders"*, Saudi Medical Journal, 2014.

Website References

****

- http://www.mgwater.com/magstory.shtml

- http://www.easy-immune-health.com/signs-of-magnesium-deficiency.html

- http://www.easy-immune-health.com/fibromyalgia-and-magnesium.html

- http://www.easy-immune-health.com/magnesium-in-pregnancy.html

- http://www.healthy.net/scr/article.aspx?ID=2060

- http://www.acatoday.org/content_css.cfm?CID=3956

- http://www.healthy.net/Health/Article/Magnesium/2060/2

- http://www.healthy.net/Health/Article/Magnesium/2060/3

- http://www.healthy.net/Health/Article/Magnesium/2060/4

- http://www.healthy.net/Health/Article/Magnesium/2060/5

- http://www.drlam.com/articles/1999-No3-MagnesiumandAging.asp

- http://www.naturalnews.com/026782_magnesium_child_children.html

- http://www.livestrong.com/article/444622-can-you-absorb-magnesium-from-epsom-salt/

- https://www.consumerlab.com/answers/What+is+the+benefit+of+magnesium+orotate+compared+to+other+forms+of+magnesium%3F/magnesium_orotate/

- http://www.mindreality.net/magnesium-supplements-can-reverse-arthritis

- http://healthblog.ivlproducts.com/blog/healthyliving/did-you-know-magnesium-deficiency-can-cause-disruptive-behaviors-in-children

- http://www.todaysgeriatricmedicine.com/archive/05 0613p30.shtml

- http://goodfoodeating.com/7341/magnesium-for-adrenal-fatigue/

- http://www.passion4health.com.au/blog/mineral-deficiencies-heavy-metal-or-toxic-mineral-excess-auto-immunity

- http://altmedicine.about.com/od/womensmenshealth/a/menstrualcramps.htm

- http://fibrocarecenter.com/2010/06/malic-acid-and-magnesium-for-fibro-pain/

- http://www.endura.com.au/articles/2009/08/magnesium-and-your-performance

- http://www.wholefoodsmagazine.com/supplements/features/reduce-high-cholesterol-nutritional-magnesium

- http://www.drdavidwilliams.com/magnsium-to-prevent-migraines/

- http://www.betterbones.com/bonenutrition/magnesium.aspx

- http://www.progressivehealth.com/thyroid-magnesium.htm

www.ingramcontent.com/pod-product-compliance
Lightning Source LLC
Chambersburg PA
CBHW030525290526
45786CB00004B/1631